The Ultimate Mediterranean Breakfast Diet Cookbook for Beginners

A Variety of Vibrant Recipes for Great Meals and Lifelong Health

Hanna Briggs

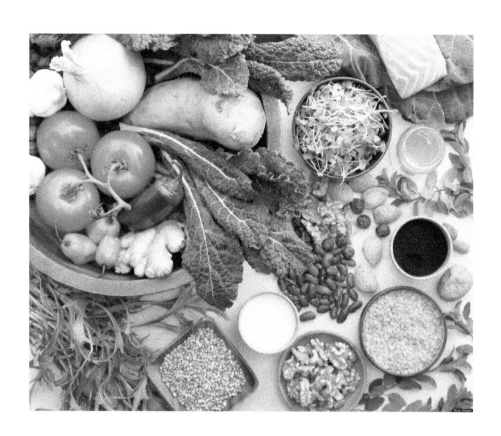

Table of contents

Introduction

Consuming the Mediterranean diet minimalizes the use of processed foods. It has been related to a reduced level of risk in developing numerous chronic diseases. It also enhances life expectancy. Several kinds of research have demonstrated many benefits in preventing cardiovascular disease, atrial fibrillation, breast cancer, and type 2 diabetes. Many pieces of evidence indicated a pattern that leads to low lipid, reduction in oxidative stress, platelet aggregation, and inflammation, and modification of growth factors and hormones involved in cancer.

Reduces Heart Diseases

According to research studies, the Mediterranean diet, which focuses on omega-3 ingredients and mono-saturated fats, reduces heart disease risk. It decreases the chances of cardiac death. The use of olive oil maintains the blood pressure levels. It is suitable for reducing hypertension. It also helps in combating the disease-promoting impacts of oxidation. This diet discourages the use of hydrogenated oils and saturated fats, which can cause heart disease.

Weight-loss

If you have been looking for diet plans for losing weight without feeling hungry, the Mediterranean diet can give you long term results. It is one of the best approaches. It is sustainable as it provides the most realistic approach to eat to feel full and energetic. This diet mostly consists of nutrient-dense food. It gives enough room for you to choose between low-carb and lower protein food. Olive oil consumed in this diet has antioxidants, natural vitamins, and some crucial fatty acids. It all improves your overall health. The Mediterranean diet focuses on natural foods, so there is very little room for junk and processed foods contributing to health-related issues and weight gain.

Most people trying the Mediterranean diet have gained positive results in cutting their weight. It is a useful option for someone looking forward to weight-loss as it provides the most unique and simple way to lose the overall calories without even changing your lifestyle that much. When you try to decrease calorie intake, losing weight is inevitable dramatically. But it will not benefit you. It will cause many health problems for you, including severe muscle loss. When you go for a Mediterranean diet, the body moves towards a sustainable model that burns calories slowly. So, it is crucial to practice the right approach and choose fat burning and more effective weight loss.

Prevents Cancer

The cornerstone of this diet is plant-based ingredients, especially vegetables and fruits. They help in preventing cancer. A plant-based diet provides antioxidants that help in protecting your DNA from damage and cell mutation. It also helps in lowering inflammation and delaying tumor growth. Various studies found that olive oil is a natural way to prevent cancer. It also decreases colon and bowel cancers. The plant-based diet balances blood sugar. It also sustains a healthy weight.

Prevents Diabetes

Numerous studies found that this healthy diet functions as an anti-inflammatory pattern, which helps fight the diseases related to chronic inflammation, Type 2 diabetes, and metabolic syndrome. It is considered very effective in preventing diabetes as it controls the insulin levels, which is a hormone to control the blood sugar levels and causes weight gain. Intake of a well-balanced diet consisting of fatty acids alongside some healthy carbohydrates and proteins is the best gift to your body. These foods help your body in burning fats more efficiently, which also provides energy. Due to the consumption of these kinds of foods, the insulin resistance level becomes non-existent, making it impossible to have high blood sugar.

Anti-aging

Choosing a Mediterranean diet without suffering from malnutrition is the most efficient and consistent anti-aging intervention. It undoubtedly expands lifespan, according to the research. The study found that the longevity biomarkers, i.e., body temperature and insulin level, and the DNA damage decreased significantly in humans by the Mediterranean diet. Other mechanisms also prove the claim made by researchers in explaining the anti-aging effects of adopting the Mediterranean diet, including reduced lipid peroxidation, high efficiency of oxidative repair, increased antioxidant defense system, and reduced mitochondrial generation rate.

Maintains Blood Sugar Level

The Mediterranean diet focuses on healthy carbs and whole grains. It has a lot of significant benefits. Consumption of whole-grain foods, like buckwheat, quinoa, and wheat berries instead of refined foods, helps you maintain blood sugar levels that ultimately gives you enough energy for the whole day.

Enhances Cognitive Health

The Mediterranean diet helps in preserving memory. It is one of the most useful steps for Alzheimer's treatment and dementia. Cognitive disorders occur when our brains do not get sufficient dopamine, which is a crucial chemical vital for mood regulation, thought processing, and body movements. Healthy fats like olive oil and nuts are good at fighting cognitive decline, mostly an age-related issue. They help counter some harmful impacts of the free radicals, inflammation, and toxins caused by having a low diet. The Mediterranean diet proves to be beneficial in decreasing

the risk of Alzheimer's to a great extent. Foods like yogurt help in having a healthy gut that improves mood, cognitive functioning, and memory.

Better Endurance Level

Mediterranean diet helps in fat loss and maintains muscle mass. It improves physical performance and enhances endurance levels. Research done on mice has shown positive results in these aspects. It also improves the health of our tissues in the long-term. The growth hormone also offers increased levels as a result of the Mediterranean diet. Which ultimately helps in improving metabolism and body composition.

Keeps You Agile

The nutrients from the Mediterranean diet reduces your risk of muscle weakness and frailty. It increases longevity. When your risk of heart disease reduces, it also reduces the risk of early death. It also strengthens your bones. Certain compounds found in olive oil help in preserving bone density. It helps increase the maturation and proliferation of the bone cells—dietary patterns of the Mediterranean diet help prevent osteoporosis.

Healthy Sleep Patterns

Our eating habits have a considerable impact on sleepiness and wakefulness. Some Mediterranean diet believers have reported an improved sleeping pattern as a result of changing their eating patterns. It has a considerable impact on your sleep because they regulate the circadian rhythm that determines our sleep patterns. If you have a regulated and balanced circadian rhythm, you will fall asleep quite quickly. You will also feel refreshed when you wake up. Another theory states that having the last meal will help you digest the food way before sleep. Digestion works best when you are upright.

Apart from focusing on plant-based eating, the Mediterranean diet philosophy emphasizes variety and moderation, living a life with perfect harmony with nature, valuing relationships in life, including sharing and enjoying meals, and having an entirely active lifestyle. The Mediterranean diet is at the crossroads. With the traditions and culture of three millennia, the Mediterranean diet lifestyle made its way to the medical world a long time ago. It has progressively recognized and became one of the successful and healthiest patterns that lead to a healthy lifestyle.

Besides metabolic, cardiovascular, cognitive, and many other benefits, this diet improves your life quality. Therefore, it is recommended today by many medical professionals worldwide. Efforts are being made in both non--Mediterranean and Mediterranean populations to make everyone benefit from the fantastic network of eating habits and patterns that began in old-time and which became a medical recommendation for a healthy lifestyle.

What to Eat and what to avoid

Fruits and vegetables: Mediterranean diet is one of the plant-based diet plans. Fresh fruits and vegetables contain a large number of vitamins, nutrients, fibers, minerals, and antioxidants

Fruits: Apple, berries, grapes, peaches, fig, grapefruit, dates, melon, oranges and pears.

Vegetables: Spinach, Brussels sprout, kale, tomatoes, kale, summer squash, onion, cauliflower, peppers, cucumbers, turnips, potatoes, sweet potatoes, and parsnips.

Seeds and nuts: Seeds and nuts are rich in monounsaturated fats and omega- 3 fatty acids.

 Seeds: pumpkin seeds, flax seeds, sesame seeds, and sunflower seeds. Nuts: Almond, hazelnuts, pistachios, cashews, and walnuts.

Whole grains: Whole grains are high in fibers and they are not processed so they do not contain unhealthy fats like trans-fats compare to processed ones.

Whole grains: Wheat, quinoa, rice, barley, oats, rye, and brown rice. You can also use bread and pasta which is made from whole grains.

Fish and seafood: Fish are the rich source of omega-3 fatty acids and proteins. Eating fish at least once a week is recommended here. The healthiest way to consume fish is to grill it. Grilling fish taste good and never need extra oil.

Fish and seafood: salmon, trout, clams, mackerel, sardines, tuna and shrimp.

Legumes: Legumes (beans) are a rich source of protein, vitamins, and fibers. Regular consumption of beans helps to reduce the risk of diabetes, cancer and heart disease.

Legumes: Kidney beans, peas, chickpeas, black beans, fava beans, lentils, and pinto beans.

Spices and herbs: Spices and herbs are used to add the taste to your meal.

Spices and herbs: mint, thyme, garlic, basil, cinnamon, nutmeg, rosemary, oregano and more.

Healthy fats: Olive oil is the main fat used in the Mediterranean diet. It helps to reduce the risk of inflammatory disorder, diabetes, cancer, and heart- related disease. It also helps to increase HDL (good cholesterol) levels and decrease LDL (bad cholesterol) levels into your body. It also helps to lose weight.

Fats: Olive oil, avocado oil, walnut oil, extra virgin olive oil, avocado, and olives.

Dairy: Moderate amounts of dairy products are allowed during the Mediterranean diet. The dairy product contains high amounts of fats.

Dairy: Greek yogurt, skim milk and cheese.

Food to avoid

Refined grains: Refined grains are not allowed in a Mediterranean diet. It raises your blood sugar level. Refined grains like white bread, white rice, and pasta.

Refined oils: Oils like vegetable oils, cottonseed oils, and soybean oils are completely avoided from the Mediterranean diet. It raises your LDL (bad cholesterol) level.

Added Sugar: Added sugar is not allowed in the Mediterranean diet. These types of artificial sugars are found in table sugar, soda, chocolate, ice cream, and candies. It raises your blood sugar level.

You should consume only natural sugars in the Mediterranean diet.

Processed foods: Generally Processed foods come in boxes. Its low-fat food should not be eaten during the diet. It contains a high amount of trans-fats. Mediterranean diet is all about to eat fresh and natural food.

Trans-fat and saturated fats: In this category of food contains butter and margarine.

Processed Meat: Mediterranean diet does not allow to use of processed meat such as bacon, hot dogs and sausage.

Breakfast recipes

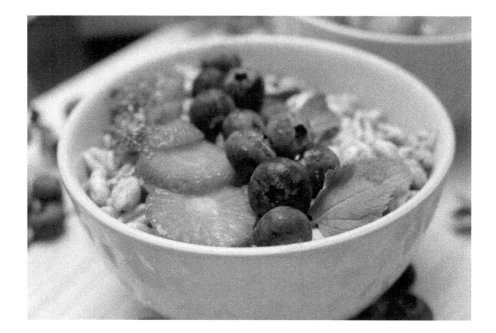

Breakfast Quesadilla
Servings: 2

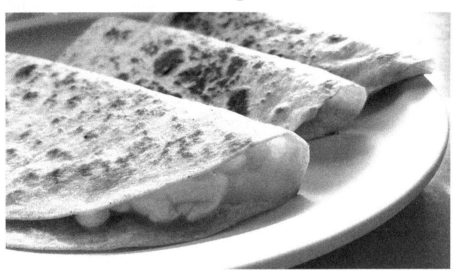

Ingredients:

- Skinless Boneless Chicken Breast
- Large Eggs
- Egg Whites
- 1 cup of Chopped Baby Spinach
- 1 tablespoon of Extra-Virgin Olive Oil
- 1/2 cup of Chopped Tomatoes
- 1/4 cup of Sour Cream
- 2/3 cup of Shredded Cheddar and Jack Cheese Blend 1 Pitted and Chopped Avocado
- 1/4 cup of Sliced Black Olives 3 Sliced Green Onions
- 2 tablespoons of Chopped Fresh Cilantro
- Salsa
- Tortillas

Directions:

Chicken:

1.   Preheat your broiler.

2. Pound your chicken breast lightly using a meat pounder.

3. Season with pepper and salt. Broil on your broiler pan for approximately 4 to 5 minutes on each side. Cook until the chicken is done and no longer pink on the inside.

4. Transfer to your chopping board and dice the chicken breast. Quesadilla:

1. Preheat your oven to 200 degrees.

2. In a bowl, whisk your eggs together.

3. Heat your oil in a frying pan over a medium heat.

4. Add your egg mixture to your pan and cook until the edges have begun to set.

5. Stir with your spatula, scraping eggs on the bottom and sides of your pan and fold them toward the center.

6. Add your spinach, chicken, and tomatoes. Continue to cook.

7. Stir frequently until your eggs are fluffy and light. Remove your pan from heat and set to the side.

8. Drizzle olive oil on a separate frying pan over a medium heat. Place a tortilla in a pan and heat up until it is warmed.

9. Flip your tortilla and sprinkle the bottom half with 1/3 cup of your cheese mixture.

10. Top your cheese with half of your egg mixture.

11. Fold your tortilla in half in your pan to cover the eggs and cheese.

12. Cook until golden brown on the bottom of tortilla.

13. Flip your quesadilla and cook the opposite side until golden brown.

14.   Transfer to your baking sheet to keep it warm while cooking your second quesadilla.

15.   Cut each into wedges. Top with cilantro, sour cream, avocado, olives, green onions, and salsa.

Hearty Breakfast Frittata w/ Tomato Salad

Servings: 4

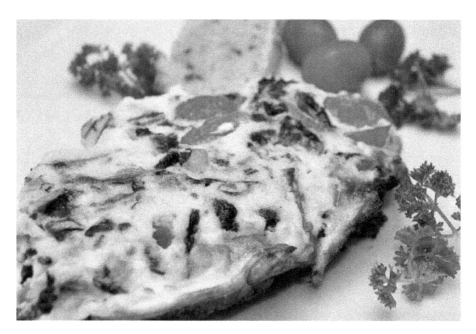

Ingredients:

- 4 Eggs
- 1 tablespoon of Vegetable Oil
- 1 2/3 pounds of Sliced and Peeled Potatoes
- 2 Onions (1 Diced / 1 Sliced Into Rings)
- 1 Small Diced Zucchini
- 1 ounce of Pitted and Sliced Black Olives
- 5 1/4 ounces of Diced Salami
- 12 ounces of Diced Tomatoes
- 1/3 cup of Whipping Cream
- 5 sprigs of Sliced Basil
- teaspoon of Balsamic Vinegar
- tablespoons of Olive Oil

Directions:

1.   Heat your vegetable oil in a pan and fry your potatoes for approximately 12 minutes.

2.   Add your onion rings, zucchini, olives, and salami. Saute for another 5 minutes.

3.   Beat your cream and eggs together. Season them and pour over the vegetables. Cover and cook over a medium heat for approximately 10 minutes.

4.   Toss together your diced onions, diced tomatoes, vinegar, olive oil, and basil. Season to taste. Slice your frittata into quarters and arrange with your tomato salad on plates.

5.   Serve and Enjoy!

Spaghetti Frittata
Servings: 6

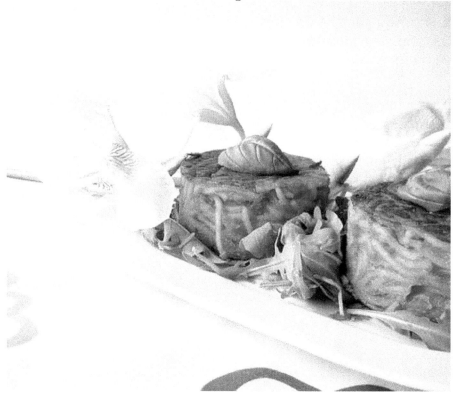

Ingredients:

- 6 Large Eggs
- 2 cups of Cooked Spaghetti 4 slices of Bacon
- 2 cloves of Minced Garlic 1 Diced Purple Onion
- 1 cup of Grated Mozzarella Cheese
- 1/4 cup of Grated Parmesan Cheese
- 3 ounces of Chopped Spinach
- 2   cloves of Minced Garlic
- 1/4 cup of Sliced Black Olives
- 6 Grape Tomatoes
- 1 tablespoon of Fresh Basil Leaves

- Ground Black Pepper
- Salt

Directions:

1.   In a big bowl, whisk your parmesan cheese and eggs until well blended. Season with pepper and salt. Add your spaghetti and toss it so everything gets combined. Set aside.

2.   Preheat your oven to 375 degrees. In a large cast iron skillet over a medium heat, cook your bacon until it is crisp and set on paper towels to drain. Add onion to your skillet and saute over a medium heat approximately 5 minutes. Stir it often until softened. Add your spinach and cook it until it has wilted. Should take 2 minutes. Add your garlic and saute until it becomes fragrant. Should take about 1 minute.

3.   Pour your spaghetti egg mixture into your skillet and sprinkle with your bacon pieces. Add your mozzarella, tomatoes, basil, and olives on top. Lower your heat and allow to cook for 3 minutes until the eggs have set on the bottom. Transfer your pan into the oven and cook for approximately 15 to 20 minutes. Remove from the oven and let it cool before serving.

4.   Serve and Enjoy!

Chickpea & Potato Hash

Servings: 4

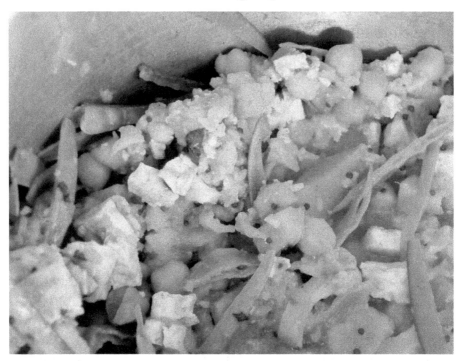

Ingredients:

- 4 cups of Frozen Shredded Hash Brown Potatoes
- 1/2 cup of Finely Chopped Onion
- 2 cups of Finely Chopped Baby Spinach
- 1 tablespoon of Minced Fresh Ginger
- 1/2 teaspoon of Salt
- 1 tablespoon of Curry Powder
- 1/4 cup of Extra-Virgin Olive Oil
- 4 Large Eggs
- 1   (15-ounce) can of Chickpeas
- 1 cup of Chopped Zucchini

Directions:

1.   Combine your spinach, potatoes, ginger, onion, salt, and curry powder in a big bowl. Heat your oil in a large sized skillet over a medium-high heat. Add in your potato mixture and press

down into a layer. Cook mixture without stirring. Cook until golden brown on bottom and crispy. Should take approximately 3 to 5 minutes.

2.   Reduce the heat to a medium-low. Fold in your zucchini and chickpeas. Once folded in, press your mixture back into an even layer. Carve 4 wells out in your mixture. Break your eggs, one at a time and slip into each of your wells. Cover and continue to cook until your eggs are set. Should take approximately 4 to 5 minutes.

3.   Serve and Enjoy!

Mediterranean Breakfast Quinoa
Servings: 4

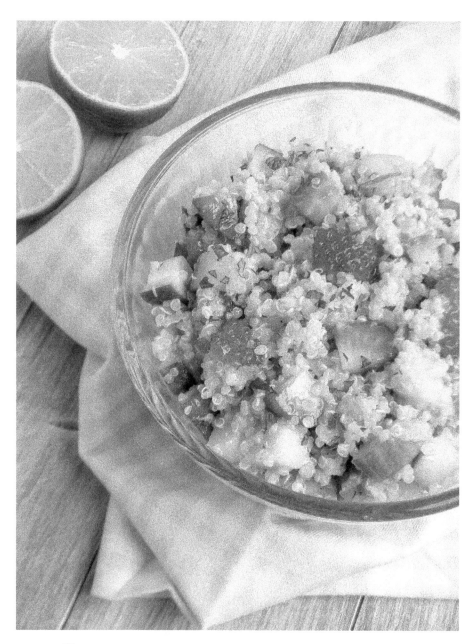

Ingredients:

- 1 teaspoon of Ground Cinnamon
- 1/4 cup of Chopped Raw Almonds
- 2 cups of Milk
- 1 cup of Quinoa
- 1 teaspoon of Vanilla Extract
- 1 teaspoon of Sea Salt
- 2 Chopped Dried Pitted Dates
- 2 tablespoons of Honey
- 5 Chopped Dried Apricots

Directions:

1.   Toast your almonds in your skillet over a medium heat. Should take approximately 3 to 5 minutes until golden. Set them aside.

2.   Heat your quinoa and cinnamon together in your saucepan over a medium heat.

3.   Add the sea salt and milk to your saucepan. Stir in well.

4.   Bring your mixture to a boil, reduce the heat to low. Cover your saucepan and allow to simmer for approximately 15 minutes.

5.   Stir in your honey, dates, vanilla, apricots, and 1/2 of your toasted almonds.

6.   Pour rest of almonds on top when ready to serve.

7.   Serve and Enjoy!

Breakfast Enchiladas
Servings: 4

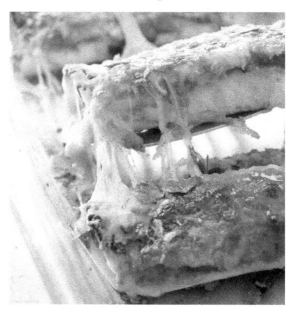

Ingredients:

- 14 Large Eggs
- 8 ounces of Spicy Vegetarian Breakfast Sausages
- 2 tablespoons of Butter
- 4 Sliced Green Onions
- 2 tablespoons of Chopped Fresh Cilantro
- 1/2 teaspoon of Pepper
- 3/4 teaspoon of Salt
- 8 Whole Wheat Tortillas
- 1 cup of Shredded Pepper Jack Cheese
- 1/3 cup of Flour
- 3 cups of Milk
- 1/3 cup of Butter
- 2 cups of Shredded Cheddar Cheese
- 4 1/2 ounces of Chopped Green Chile
- 1/2 cup of Grape Tomatoes

- 1/8 cup of Sliced Black Olives

Directions:

1.   Melt your butter in a saucepan over a medium heat. Whisk in the flour until it is smooth. Cook, constantly whisking for approximately 1 minute. Gradually, whisk in your milk and continue to cook over a medium heat. Whisk constantly until mixture has thickened. Should take approximately 5 minutes. Remove from heat. Whisk in your chile, cheddar cheese, and salt.

2.   Cook your sausage. Remove from pan when finished. Drain if necessary.

3.   Melt butter in a large skillet over a medium heat. Add in your cilantro and green onions. Saute them. Add your salt, eggs, and pepper. Cook without any stirring until your eggs have begun to set. Bring your spatula across the bottom of your pan to help distribute uncooked eggs. Keep cooking until the eggs have gotten thick but are still moist. Remove from the heat and fold in your sausage and 1 1/2 cups of cheese sauce from the first step.

4.   Spoon 1/3 of a cup of your egg mixture down the center of each of your tortillas and roll up. Place the seam side down in a greased 13 x 9 baking dish. Repeat for all your tortillas. Pour your remaining cheese mixture over the tortillas evenly and sprinkle with pepper jack cheese. Refrigerate approximately 45 minutes.

5.   Bake at 350 degrees for approximately 30 minutes or until your cheese is bubbling. Sprinkle with the toppings of your choice.

6.   Serve and Enjoy!

Mediterranean Breakfast Wraps
Servings: 4

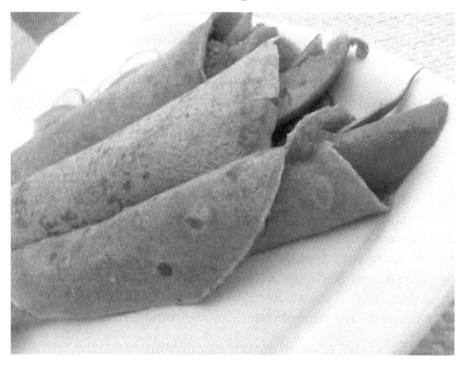

Ingredients:

- 4 Eggs
- 4 Tortillas
- 1 tablespoon of Water
- 1/2 teaspoon of Garlic Chipotle Seasoning
- 4 tablespoons of Crumbled Feta Cheese
- 4 tablespoons of Tomato Chutney
- cup of Chopped Fresh Spinach Leaves
- Dried Tomatoes
- Bacon
- Prosciutto
- Salt
- Pepper

Directions:

1. Mix your eggs, seasoning, and water.

2. Heat a skillet. Add some butter or bacon grease. Add in your egg mixture and scramble for 3 to 4 minutes until cooked.

3. Lay your tortillas out and divide your eggs among them evenly. Leave the edges free so you can fold them.

4. Top each layer of your eggs with an even amount of cheese. Approximately 1 tablespoon for each wrap.

5. Add tomato chutney. Approximately 1 tablespoon for each wrap.

6. Add spinach. Approximately 1/4 cup for each wrap.

7. Add bacon and prosciutto. I use a couple of slices on each wrap but feel free to add the amount you prefer.

8. Roll up the tortillas burrito style. Be sure to fold in both of your ends.

9. Cook approximately 1 minute on a skillet or panini maker.

10. Serve and Enjoy!

Panera Mediterranean Breakfast Sandwich
Servings: 1

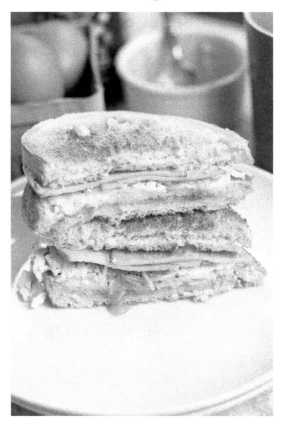

Ingredients:

- 2   Egg Whites
- 1 Ciabatta Roll
- 1 slice of Tomato
- 1 slice of White Cheddar Cheese
- 1 tablespoon of Pesto
- 1 handful of Baby Spinach
- Cracked Black Pepper

Directions:

1.   Split your roll and place the cheese on bottom half.

2.   Lightly broil the half of roll with cheese on it in your toaster oven.

3.   Spray a ramekin or mug with cooking spray. Pour eggs whites into it and cover. Microwave for approximately 45 to 60 seconds. Place tomato slice on top of your cooked egg and microwave it for about 10 more seconds.

4.   Place your cooked egg and tomato on top of your cheese covered half of roll. Sprinkle the top with cracked pepper. Spread pesto on the top half of your roll. Add spinach on top of the tomato and put your sandwich together.

5.   Serve and Enjoy!

Mediterranean Eggs

Servings: 4

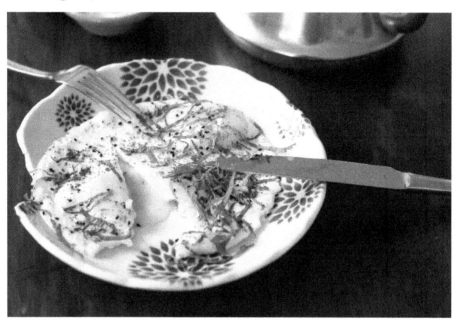

Ingredients:

- 8 Large Eggs

- 5 Yellow Onions

- 1 tablespoon of Extra-Virgin Olive Oil

- 1 tablespoon of Butter

- 1 clove of Minced Garlic

- 1/3 cup of Sun Dried Tomatoes

- 3 ounces of Feta Cheese Kosher Salt

- Ground Black Pepper Chopped Parsley (optional)

- Ciabatta Rolls (optional)

Directions:

1.   Heat butter and oil in a steel skillet over a medium heat. Once your butter has melted add in your onions and stir to coat with oil and butter.

2.   Reduce the heat so your onions barely sizzle. Allow onions to cook for about an hour until they are a deep brown color and soft. Stir every 5 to 10 minutes.

3.   Add your garlic and tomatoes. Cook and stir for 1 to 3 minutes until fragrant. Arrange your mixture into an even layer on your pan and crack your eggs over the top. Sprinkle with salt, pepper, and crumbled feta cheese. Cover it with a tight lid and let cook approximately 10 to 15 minutes undisturbed.

4.   Remove from the heat once your eggs are cooked to your desired level. Add optional ingredients if you want.

5.   Serve and Enjoy!

Mediterranean Breakfast Casserole

Servings: 8

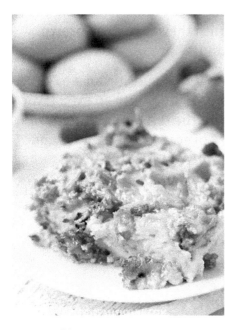

Ingredients:

- 8 Large Eggs

- 4 Large Egg Whites

- 1 tablespoon of Fresh Grated Parmesan Cheese

- 1/4 cup of Almond Milk

- 1 tablespoon of Chopped Oregano

- 1/4 teaspoon of Ground Pepper

- 1 teaspoon of Sea Salt

- 1/2 cup of Crumbled Feta Cheese

- 1/4 teaspoon of Garlic Powder

- 4 ounces of Baby Spinach
- 4 Artichoke Hearts
- 1/2 cup of Green Onions
- 2 Diced Roma Tomatoes
- 2 Minced Garlic Cloves
- 2/3 cup of Sliced Mushrooms

Directions:

1. Preheat your oven to 375 degrees.

2. In your mixing bowl, whisk together egg whites, eggs, salt, oregano, garlic powder, and pepper. Mix in your feta cheese and set to the side.

3. Spray a 9 x 13 baking dish with your cooking spray. In your dish, layer your green onions, tomatoes, artichokes, spinach, garlic, and mushrooms. Pour the egg mixture over your vegetables. Shake your casserole dish to distribute your egg mixture evenly.

4. Bake for approximately 30 minutes. Allow to rest for 10 minutes before cutting into it.

5. Serve and Enjoy!

Mediterranean Egg White Breakfast Sandwich
Servings: 4

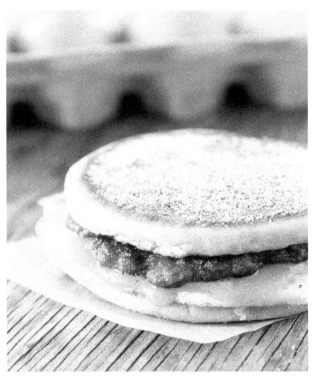

Ingredients:

- 1/4 cup of Egg Whites

- 10 ounces of Grape Tomatoes 1 teaspoon of Butter

- 1 teaspoon of Parsley

- Whole Grain Ciabatta Roll

- 1 tablespoon of Pesto

- slices of Muenster Cheese

- tablespoon of Extra-Virgin Olive Oil

- Black Pepper

- Kosher Salt

Directions:

1.   Make your roasted tomatoes. Preheat your oven to 400 degrees. Slice your tomatoes in half. Place them on a baking sheet and drizzle with your olive oil. Toss the tomatoes to coat. Season with pepper and salt. Roast in the oven for approximately 20 minutes. Skins should appear wrinkled once ready.

2.   Melt your butter over a medium heat in a small skillet. Pour in the egg whites and season them with pepper and salt. Sprinkle parsley on top. Cook approximately 3 to 4 minutes until the egg is done. Be sure to flip it at least once.

3.   Toast your ciabatta roll. Cut in half and spread both halves with the pesto once toasted. Place your egg on the bottom half of the sandwich. Top with cheese. Add your roasted tomatoes and the top half of the roll.

4.   Serve and Enjoy!

Mediterranean Scramble

Servings: 1

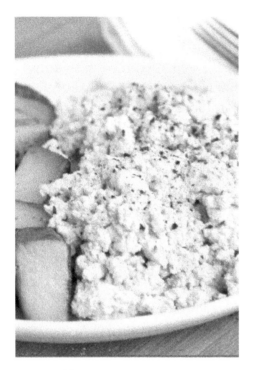

Ingredients:

- 2   Eggs
- 1/4 cup of Chopped Baby Spinach
- 2 tablespoons of Crumbled Feta Cheese
- 2 tablespoons of Diced Zucchini
- 1 tablespoon of Milk Butter
- Ground Pepper
- Salt

Directions:

1.   In your medium sized bowl, whisk together milk and eggs until they are combined. Heat a pan over a medium-low heat. Add enough butter to coat the bottom of your pan. Once the butter has melted, add your eggs.

2.   Once eggs begin to set, use your spatula and move eggs inward toward the center of your pan. Continue around outside of your pan in the same way.

3.   As curds begin to form, add your zucchini, feta, and spinach to your eggs. Mix well to combine. Move the eggs around your pan until they become fully set.

4.   Move eggs onto your plate and season with pepper and salt.

5.   Serve and Enjoy!

Moroccan Style Poached Eggs

Servings: 3

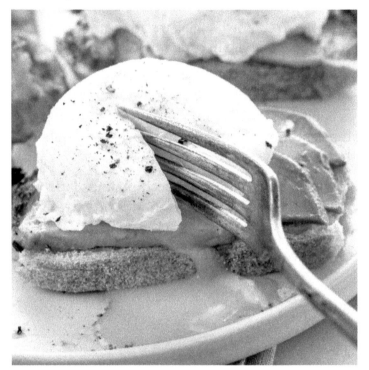

Ingredients:

- 3 Large Eggs

- 1 tablespoon of Olive Oil

- 1 clove of Grated Garlic

- 1/4 cup of Chopped Leeks

- 1 1/2 tablespoons of Tomato Paste

- 1 1/4 cups of Chopped Tomatoes

- 1/2 teaspoon of Black Pepper

- 1/2 teaspoon of Ground Cumin

- 1/4 teaspoon of Salt

- 1 teaspoon of Paprika

- tablespoon of Chopped Cilantro Pinch of Sugar

Directions:

1.　　Heat olive oil in your pan. Once hot, saute your grated garlic, chopped leeks, and 1/4 cup of water on medium-low heat and allow to simmer for about 5 to 10 minutes.

2.　　Add your chopped tomatoes, tomato paste, salt, sugar, pepper, spices and allow to simmer for another 5 to 10 minutes.

3.　　You can adjust the consistency of your sauce by adding 1 to 2 tablespoons of water as needed. Be sure to keep a lid on the pan while simmering.

4.　　Crack your eggs into the sauce. Cover your pan and poach your eggs approximately 5 to 6 minutes until the eggs are set well.

5.　　Season with pepper and salt. Garnish with your chopped cilantro. You can also add the toasted bread of your choice on the side. Allow to rest 5 minutes before serving.

6.　　Serve and Enjoy!

Healthy Mediterranean Veggie Omelette

Servings: 1

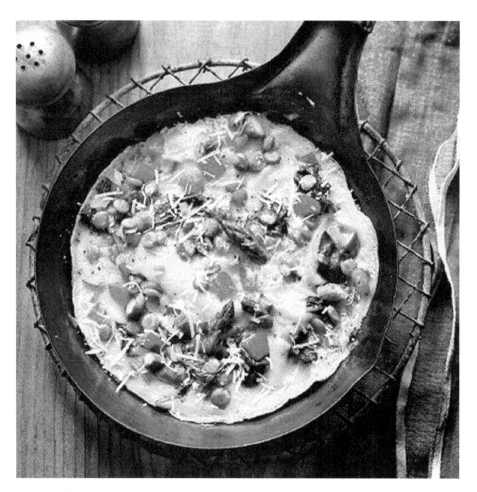

Ingredients:

- 2   eggs
- 1/3 cup of Baby Spinach
- 1/3 cup of Grape Tomatoes
- 1/3 cup of Sliced Crimini Mushrooms

- 1/4 cup of Feta Cheese

- 2 tablespoons of Mediterranean Spice Seasoning

- Extra-Virgin Olive Oil

Directions:

1.   In a mixing bowl, whisk your 2 eggs together.

2.   Pour into a small sized frying pan and cook over a medium heat for approximately 2 minutes.

3.   Add your vegetables and seasoning.

4.   Once eggs are set and solid, fold them in half.

5.   Serve and Enjoy!

Greek Omelet

Servings: 2

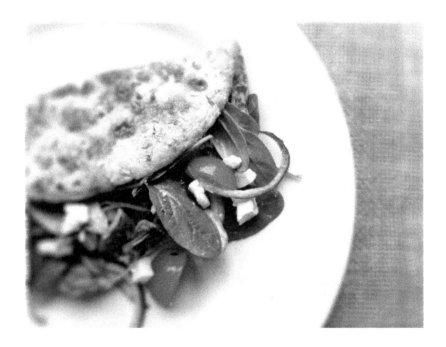

Ingredients:

- 4 Large Eggs
- 1/4 cup of Cooked Spinach
- 1/2 cup of Crumbled Feta Cheese
- 2 tablespoons of Chopped Fresh Dill
- 2 Thinly Sliced Scallions
- 2 teaspoons of Extra-Virgin Olive Oil Ground Pepper

Directions:

1.   Squeeze your spinach to remove any of the excess water. Blend your eggs with a fork in your bowl. Add scallions, feta, pepper, spinach, and dill. Gently mix them together with your rubber spatula.

2.   Preheat your broiler. Place a rack about 4 inches away from the heat source.

3.   Heat your oil in a skillet over a medium heat. Pour your egg mixture into the skillet and tilt it to distribute it evenly. Reduce your heat to a medium-low and cook mixture until the bottom has turned a light golden color. Be sure to lift up the edges to allow any uncooked eggs to flow in underneath. Should take approximately 3 to 4 minutes.

4.   Place your pan under your broiler and cook egg mixture until the top has set. This should take an additional 1 to 3 minutes.

5.   Remove omelet from pan and cut into wedges.

6.   Serve and Enjoy!

Greek Scramble

Servings: 4

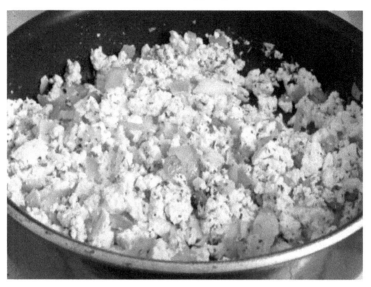

Ingredients:

- 10 Large Eggs
- 1/4 cup of Milk
- 2/3 cup of Crumbled Feta Cheese
- 1/2 teaspoon of Fine Salt
- 1 tablespoon of Olive Oil
- 1/4 teaspoon of Ground Black Pepper
- 6 ounces of Baby Spinach
- 1/2 Diced Yellow Onion
- 1 cup of Quartered Cherry Tomatoes
- Pita Bread

Directions:

1.   Whisk your eggs, salt, pepper, and milk in a large bowl. Set to the side.

2.   Heat your oil in a skillet over a medium heat until simmering. Add your onion. Stir occasionally, cook approximately 5 minutes. Add the spinach, tossing until completely wilted and no liquid is left. Should take approximately 3 minutes.

3.   Reduce your heat to a medium-low and pour in your egg mixture. Cook for 2 minutes. Using a rubber spatula, push your set eggs from the edge of the skillet to the center. Spread your uncooked eggs back into an even layer. Repeat, pushing the set eggs from edges to the center every 30 seconds until they are all nearly set. Total cooking time should be approximately 6 minutes.

4.   Remove skillet from the heat and fold in your tomatoes. Toast your pita bread.

5.   Serve and Enjoy!

Cheesy Mediterranean Scramble
Servings: 6

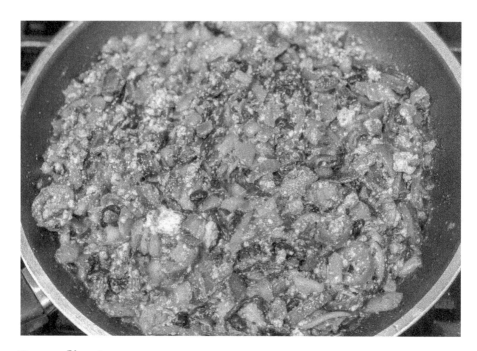

Ingredients:

- 6 slices of Whole Wheat Bread
- 3 cartons of Egg Substitute
- 1/8 teaspoon of Ground Black Pepper
- 1/2 teaspoon of Crushed Dried Basil Leaves
- 1 1/2 tablespoons of Butter Spread
- 2 tablespoons of Low Fat Feta Cheese
- 1 Small Chopped Red Pepper
- 1 Small Chopped Sweet Onion

Directions:

1.   In a large bowl add egg substitute, black pepper, and basil. Whisk and set aside.

2.   In a 10-inch skillet, melt your butter spread over a medium-high heat and cook your onion and red pepper. Stir occasionally for 4 minutes until the vegetables get tender. Stir in your egg mixture and allow it to set slightly.

3.   Cook eggs until set, stirring occasionally. Sprinkle with cheese. Toast your slices of white bread.

4.   Serve and Enjoy!

Mediterranean Omelet
Servings: 4

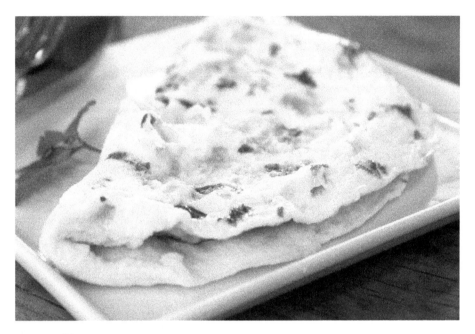

Ingredients:

- 2 Large Eggs
- 1 Tomato
- 1 teaspoon of Olive Oil
- 3 sprigs of Chives
- 4 1/4 tablespoons of Feta Cheese
- 1/2 teaspoon of Dried Oregano Olives
- Pinch of Salt

Directions:

1.   In frying pan heat your olive oil.

2.   Add your chopped tomato, oregano, and onion. Cook until the tomatoes are no longer soft.

3.   Add in your olives and turn the heat off. Add your feta cheese.

4.   In a different frying pan add add your eggs and salt and cook.

5.   Combine ingredients and add your toppings.

6.   Serve and Enjoy

Huevos Revueltos

Servings: 4

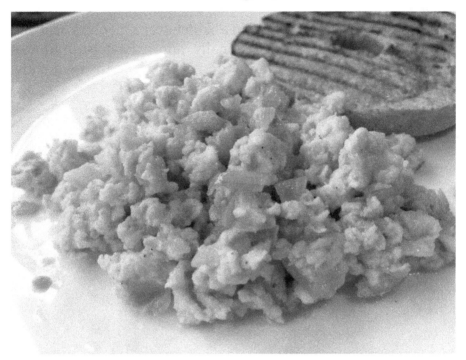

Ingredients:

- 4 Eggs
- 2 tablespoons of Butter Spread
- 1/4 cup of Crumbled Queso Fresco Cheese
- 1/2 cup of Chopped Tomatoes
- 1/2 cup of Chopped Onion
- Chopped Fresh Cilantro

Directions:

1.   Melt your butter spread in a skillet over a medium heat and add your vegetables. Stir occasionally, approximately 4 minutes or until they are tender. Add in your eggs. Stir frequently, approximately 2 minutes until the eggs are done.

2.   Sprinkle with your cilantro and cheese.

3.   Serve and Enjoy!

Creamy Cuban Fu Fu
Servings: 8

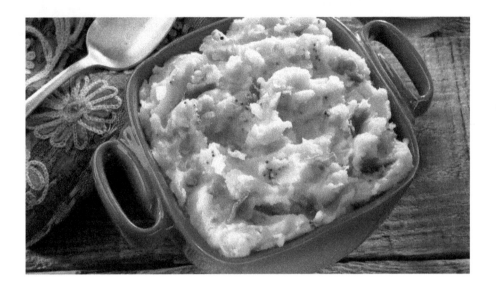

Ingredients:

- 4 slices of Chopped Bacon
- 4 Sliced Sweet Plantains
- 1 Small Chopped Onion
- 1/2 cup of Light Mayonnaise
- 1 clove of Chopped Garlic

Directions:

1.   Cover your plantains with water in a 4-quart sauce skillet. Bring the skillet to a boil over a medium-high heat. Reduce the heat and allow to simmer for approximately 10 minutes until the plantains are tender. Drain the water from your skillet and mash your plantains. Set to the side.

2.   Cook your bacon in a 10-inch skillet over a medium heat until the bacon is crisp. Drain excess liquid. Reserve a tablespoon of the bacon drippings.

3.   Heat your reserved drippings in the same skillet and cook your onion approximately 4 minutes. Make sure to occasionally stir. Once the onion is tender, add your garlic and cook approximately 1 more minute.

4.   Combine your plantains, onion mixture, 1/2 of the bacon, and mayonnaise in a serving bowl. Garnish it with your remaining bacon.

5.   Serve and Enjoy!

Roasted Asparagus Prosciutto & Egg
Servings: 4

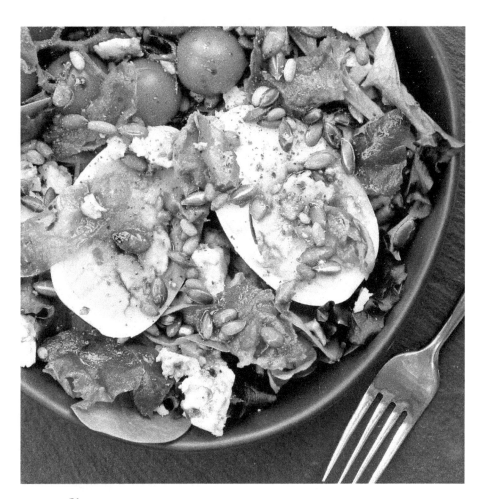

Ingredients:

- 1 bunch of Trimmed Fresh Asparagus
- 1 tablespoon of Olive Oil
- 1 tablespoon of Extra-Virgin Olive Oil

- 2 ounces of Minced Prosciutto
- 4 Eggs
- 1 teaspoon of Distilled White Vinegar
- 1/2 of a Lemon (Juiced & Zested)
- Pinch of Ground Black Pepper
- Pinch of Salt

Directions:

1. Preheat your oven to 425 degrees.

2. Place your asparagus in a baking dish and then drizzle with your extra-virgin olive oil.

3. Heat olive oil in your skillet over a medium-low heat. Add in your prosciutto. Cook approximately 3 to 4 minutes. Stir it until

it is golden colored and rendered. Sprinkle your oil and prosciutto over your asparagus. Season with your pepper and toss it to coat well.

4. Roast it in your oven for approximately 10 minutes. Take out and toss it again.

5. Place back in your oven for an additional 5 minutes until asparagus is firm yet still tender.

6. Fill a big saucepan with approximately 2 to 3 inches of water and boil over a high heat. Reduce the heat to medium-low. Pour in your vinegar and salt.

7.   Crack egg into a bowl and then slip your egg gently into the water. Continue this with all of your remaining eggs. Poach your eggs until the whites are firm and the yolks have gotten thick but not hard. Should take approximately 4 to 6 minutes.

8.   Remove your eggs using a slotted spoon. Dab on a towel to help remove any excess water. Move to a warm plate.

9.   Drizzle lemon juice over asparagus. Place asparagus on plate and top with your poached egg and a pinch of the lemon zest. Season it with your black pepper.

10.   Serve and Enjoy!

Creamy Loaded Mashed Potatoes
Servings: 8

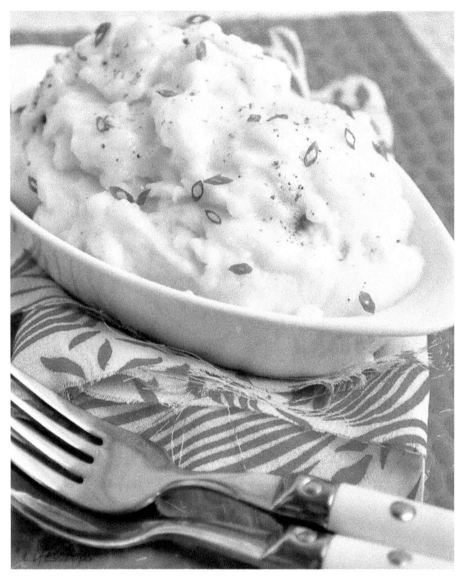

Ingredients:

- 3 pounds of Cubed and Peeled Potatoes

- 1 cup of Mayonnaise
- 1 cup of Sour Cream
- 6 slices of Bacon or Turkey Bacon
- 1 1/2 cups of Shredded Cheddar Cheese
- 3 Chopped Green Onions

Directions:

1. Cover your potatoes with water in a 4-quart sauce skillet. Boil over a high heat. Reduce heat to low and cook approximately 10 minutes until the potatoes are tender. Drain them and mash.

2. Preheat your oven to 375 degrees. Spray baking dish with cooking spray.

3. Stir in mayonnaise, green onions, 4 strips of crumbled bacon, and sour cream. Turn them into your baking dish and cook approximately 30 minutes.

4. Top with remaining 1/2 cup of cheese and your bacon. Bake for 5 more minutes until the cheese has melted.

5. Serve and Enjoy!

Greek Yogurt w/ Berries & Seeds
Servings: 1

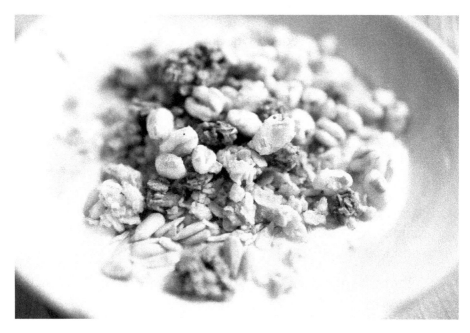

Ingredients:

- 1 handful of Blueberries 1 handful of Raspberries
- 1 tablespoon of Greek Yogurt
- 1 teaspoon of Sunflower Seeds
- 1 teaspoon of Pumpkin Seeds 1
- teaspoon of Sliced Almonds

Directions:

1.   Wash and dry your berries. Place them into a dish.

2.   Spoon your Greek yogurt on top and sprinkle with your seeds and nuts.

3.   Serve and Enjoy!

Greek Yogurt Parfait
Servings: 4

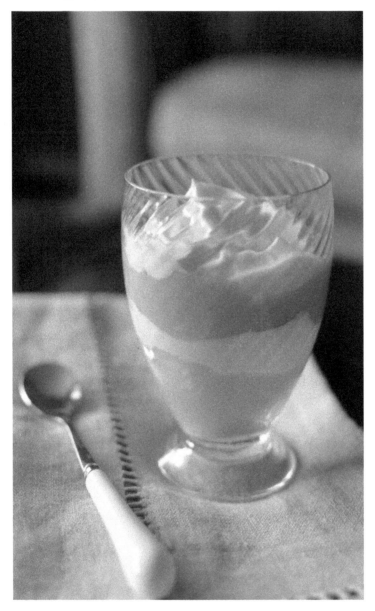

Ingredients:

- 4 teaspoons of Honey

- 3 cups of Plain Fat-Free Greek Yogurt
- 28 Clementine Segments
- 1 teaspoon of Vanilla Extract
- 1/4 cup of Shelled Unsalted Dry Roasted Chopped Pistachios

Directions:

1.   Combine your vanilla and Greek yogurt in your bowl. Spoon

in 1/3 cup of your yogurt mixture into 4 parfait glasses. Top each of them with 1/2 teaspoon of honey, 1/2 tablespoon of nuts, and 5 clementine sections.

2.   Top your parfaits with remaining yogurt mixture. Top each with 1/2 teaspoon of honey, 1/2 tablespoon of nuts, and 2 clementine segments.

3.   Serve and Enjoy!

Waffled Falafel
Servings: 4

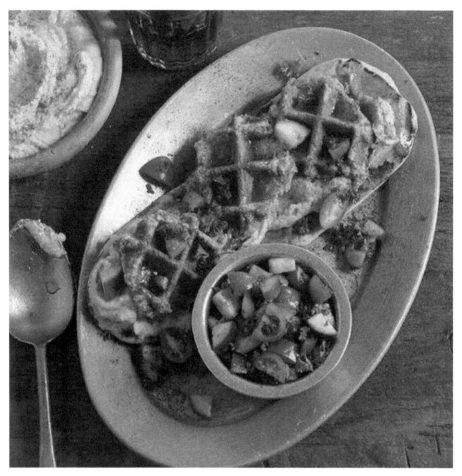

Ingredients:

- 2 cans of Garbanzo Beans
- 1 Chopped Medium Onion
- 2 Large Egg Whites
- 1/4 cup of Chopped Fresh Cilantro

- 1/4 cup of Chopped Fresh Parsley
- 1 1/2 tablespoons of All Purpose Flour
- 3 Cloves of Roasted Garlic
- 2 teaspoons of Ground Cumin
- 1 3/4 teaspoons of Salt
- 1 teaspoon of Ground Coriander
- 1/4 teaspoon of Cayenne Pepper
- 1/4 teaspoon of Ground Black Pepper
- Pinch of Ground Cardamom
- Cooking Spray

Directions:

1. Preheat your waffle iron. Spray inside of iron with your cooking spray.

2. Process your garbanzo beans in your food processor until they are coarsely chopped.

3. Add in your egg whites, onion, parsley, cilantro, flour, garlic, cumin, coriander, salt, cayenne pepper, black pepper and ground cardamom to your garbanzo beans.

4. Pulse in your food processor until your batter resembles a coarse meal. Scrap down the sides while pulsing.

5. Pour your batter into a bowl and stir it with your fork.

6. Spoon 1/4 cup of batter onto each section of your waffle iron. Cook until they are evenly browned. Should take approximately 5 minutes. Repeat process with batter until it has all been used.

7. Serve and Enjoy!

Honey-Caramelized Figs with Greek Yogurt
Servings: 4

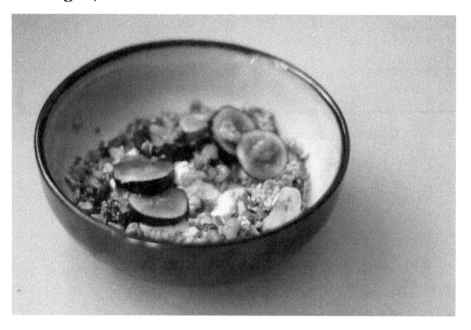

Ingredients:

- Four fresh halved figs
- Two tablespoons of melted butter, 30ml
- Two tablespoons of brown sugar, 30ml
- Two cups of Greek yogurt 500ml
- 1/4 cup of honey, 60ml

Directions

1. Take a non-stick skillet and preheat it over a medium flame

2. Put the butter on the pan and toss the figs into it and sprinkle in some brown sugar over it.

3. Put the figs on the pan and cut off the side of the figs.

4. Cook the figs on a medium flame for 2-3 minutes until they turns a golden brown.

5. Turn over the figs and cook them for 2-3 minutes again

6. Remove the figs from the pan and let it cool down a little.

7. Take a plate and put a scoop of Greek yogurt on it. Put the cooked figs over the yogurts and drizzle the honey over it.

Greek Quinoa Breakfast Bowl
Servings: 2

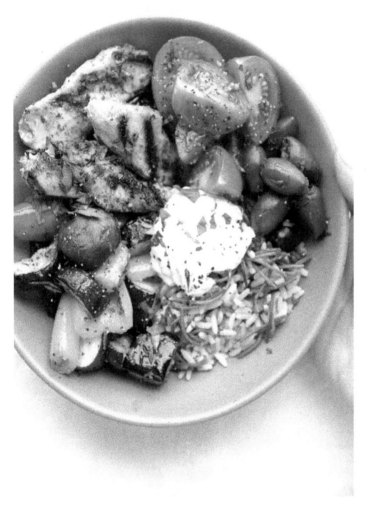

Ingredients:

- 2 large eggs

- 3/4 cup Greek yogurt
- 2   cups of cooked quinoa
- 3/4 cup muhammara
- 3   ounces of baby spinach
- 4   ounces of marinated kalamata olives
- 6 ounces of sliced cherry tomatoes
- 1 halved lemon hot chili oil
- salt & pepper to taste
- fresh dill and sesame seeds to garnish

Directions

1.   Add all the ingredients, Greek yogurt, granulated garlic, onion powder, salt, and pepper and whisk them all together and set aside.

2.   In a different large saucepan, heat the olive oil on medium-high

heat and add the spinach. You have to keep in mind to cook the spinach till it is slightly wilted. This takes about 3-4 minutes.

3.   After that, cook the cherry tomatoes in the same skillet for 3-4 minutes till they are softened.

4.   Stir in the egg mixture into this for about 7 to 9 minutes, until it has set and cook them so that they get scrambled.

5.	After the eggs have set, stir in the quinoa and feta and cook until it is heated all the way through and serve it hot with some fresh dill and sesame seeds to garnish.

Date and Walnut Overnight Oats
Servings: 2

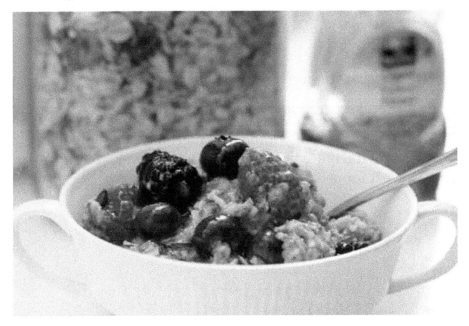

Ingredients:

- 1/3 cup of yogurt
- 2/3 cup of oats
- cup of milk
- tsp date syrup or you can also use maple syrup or honey 1
- mashed banana
- ¼ tsp cinnamon
- ¼ cup walnuts
- pinch of salt (approx.1/8 tsp)

Directions

1.   Firstly, get a mason jar or a small bowl and add all the ingredients.

2.   After that stir and mix all the ingredients well.

3.   Cover it securely and cool it in a refrigerator overnight.

4.   After that, take it out the next morning, add more liquid or cinnamon if required and serve cold. (However, you can also microwave it for people with a warmer palate.)

Pastry-Less Spanakopita
Servings: 4

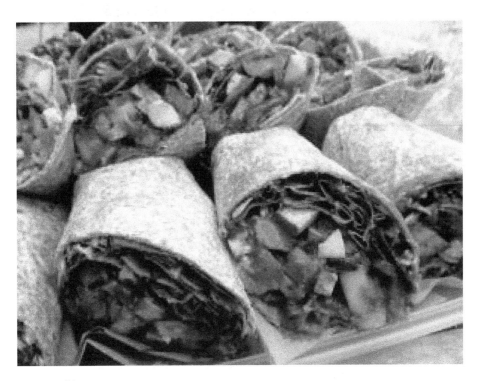

Ingredients:

- 1/8 teaspoons black pepper, add as per taste

- 1/3 cup of Extra virgin olive oil

- 4 lightly beaten eggs

- 7 cups of Lettuce, preferably a spring mix (mesclun)

- 1/2 cup of crumbled Feta cheese

- 1/8 teaspoon of Sea salt, add to taste

- 1 finely chopped medium Yellow onion

Directions

1.   For this delicious recipe, you need to first start by preheating the oven to 180C and grease the flan dish.

2.   Once done, pour the extra virgin olive oil into a large saucepan and heat it over medium heat with the onions, until they are translucent. To that, add greens and keep stirring until all the ingredients are wilted.

3.   After completing that, you should season it with salt and pepper and transfer the greens to the prepared dish and sprinkle on some feta cheese.

4.   Pour the eggs and bake it for 20 minutes till it is cooked through and slightly brown.

Apricot Marmalade
Servings: 4

Ingredients:

- 3 kilograms of Firm Apricots
- 1 glass of Water
- glass of Lemon Juice
- 2250 grams of Sugar

Directions:

1.　　Wash your apricots and remove their pits.

2.　　Place them in layers in your skillet, alternating a layer of apricots, a layer of sugar, a layer of apricots, a layer of sugar etc. Pour water on top.

3.　　Place your skillet over a low heat and stir until all the sugar has dissolved.

4.　　Adjust heat to simmer your marmalade.

5.　　Stir constantly using a wooden ladle so your marmalade doesn't stick to your skillet.

6.　　Cook the mixture until it gets shiny and transparent.

7.　　Once marmalade is thick, add your lemon juice and allow to boil.

8.　　Move off the burner and allow to cool. Place it in jars. Seal jars to preserve your marmalade.

9.　　Serve and Enjoy!

Yogurt Cheese
Servings: 2

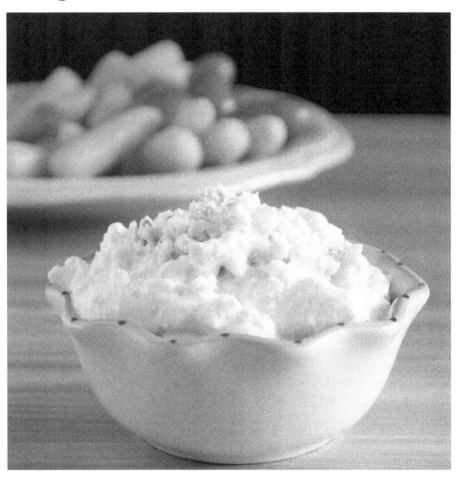

Ingredients:

- 4 cups full-fat plain yogurt
- teaspoon unrefined sea salt
- extra-virgin olive oil, unfiltered

Directions:

1.   Using a spatula, scrape the yogurt into the lined strainer. Fold the ends of the cheesecloth over the yogurt and refrigerate overnight, or for a minimum of 12 hours.

2.   Remove the thickened strained cheese from the cloth. Transfer

the mixture to a shallow serving dish and smooth out the top in a circular fashion using a spatula.

3.   Make a few swirls in the, then drizzle a fairly generous amount of olive oil in the indentations.

4.   Sprinkle with e olives in the middle. Serve with bread for dipping.

Omelet Provencale
Servings: 4

Ingredients:

- 2 teaspoons for serving extra-virgin olive oil
- 2 zucchini, diced
- 2 roasted red peppers from a jar, drained, chopped finely
- 1 clove garlic, chopped finely
- ¼ cup chives, finely chopped
- 8 eggs
- ½ teaspoon unrefined sea salt or salt
- ¼ teaspoon freshly ground black pepper
- ½ cup goat cheese
- 2 tablespoons fresh basil, chopped finely
- 4 cups mixed field greens such as baby spinach or arugula
- 1 teaspoon lemon juice

Directions:

1. Heat 2 tablespoons (30 ml) of the oil in a large skillet over medium heat. Add the zucchini, roasted red pepper, garlic, and chives, then cook gently for about 10 minutes, until softened.

2.   Break the eggs into a bowl, whisk lightly and season with salt and pepper. Pour the eggs into the skillet, turn, and swivel to coat. Add knobs of the goat cheese over the top and sprinkle with basil.

3.   Serve a slice of the omelet on the side.

Chili Cheese Omelet

Servings: 4

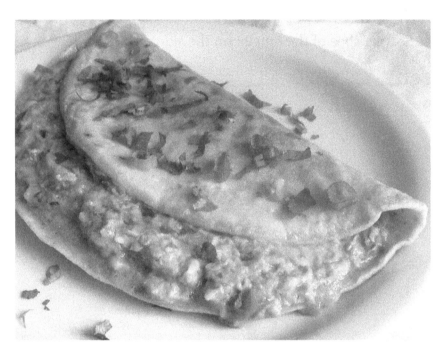

Ingredients:

- 2 Tbsp. green chilis, chopped 1 large green onion, chopped

- 2 tbsp. olive oil

- 2   oz. Monterey Jack cheese, grated optional garnish

- sour cream salt

- pepper to taste

Directions:

1.   Make an individual omelet according to instructions. When the eggs are nearly set, and just moist on top, quickly spread the grated cheese over one side of the omelet.

2.   Sprinkle the chopped green onions and green chilis evenly over the cheese and fold the other side of the omelet over the filling. Leave the omelet in the pan, on medium-low heat, for another minute or so, just long enough for the cheese to melt.

3.   Slide the omelet onto a warmed plate and serve immediately, garnished with sour cream if desired.

Cream of Carrot and Potato Soup
Servings: 4

Ingredients:

- 3 cups carrots, sliced
- 2 potatoes, diced
- 1 yellow onion, chopped
- 4 Tbs. flour
- ½ cup olive oil
- 1 tsp. sugar
- ½ cup water
- 1½ cups light cream
- 4½ cups milk paprika
- cayenne pepper
- 1 clove garlic, minced (optional)
- Brandy garnish
- 1 tsp. salt
- fresh-ground black pepper chopped parsley, for garnish

Directions:

1. Sauté the carrots and onions in a large skillet or soup skillet in 4 tablespoons of olive oil for a few minutes. Add the

sugar, 1 tsp. salt, the diced potato, and the water. Cover tightly and simmer until the vegetables are just tender.

2.   Purée the vegetables in a blender with the cream.

3.   Melt the remaining 4 tablespoons butter in a skillet and stir in the flour. Cook the roux until it is golden. Heat the milk and stir

it into the roux with a whisk. Cook the white sauce over a very small flame, stirring often, until it is thickened.

4.   Combine the carrot purée and the white sauce in a large skillet. Grate in some pepper and add paprika and cayenne to taste, as well as a little minced garlic if you like. Add a little brandy and salt to taste.

5.   Simmer the soup gently for another 10 or 15 minutes, stirring occasionally. Serve hot, garnished with chopped parsley.

Lima Bean Salad

Servings: 2

Ingredients:

2   cups dry lima beans, large

⅓ cup olive oil 1½ qts. water

¼ cup white wine vinegar salt

fresh-ground black pepper

Directions:

1.   Put the beans in a large skillet with the water and 1 teaspoon salt, bring to a boil, and then reduce the flame. Simmer the beans gently for about 1 hour, or until they are just tender. Drain them while they are still hot, reserving the liquid.

2.   In a skillet, boil the bean liquid vigorously for a few minutes until it is substantially thickened. Measure out ⅔ cup of the thickened liquid into a bowl.

3.   Add 1 tablespoon salt plus all of the other ingredients to the warm liquid and whisk until well blended and you have a smooth sauce.

4.   Pour the sauce over the beans while they are still warm and mix them up gently with a wooden spoon, being careful not to mash them. Refrigerate for several hours.

5.   Before serving, stir the salad again so that all the beans are well coated with the dressing.

Mushrooms and Watercress Salad

Servings: 2

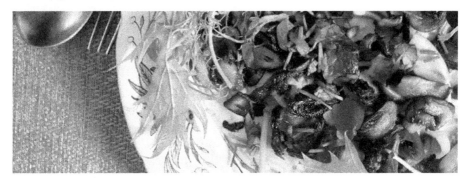

Ingredients:

8 firm mushrooms, sliced 4 eggs, hard-boiled

1 bunch watercress

½ medium-sized red onion 1 lb. string beans

1 medium-small cucumber

¾ cup Sour Cream Dressing

½ cup mayonnaise

Directions:

1.   Peel and dice the skillet to, cook it in boiling salted water until it is tender, drain, and run cold water over it until it is cool. Put it in the refrigerator.

2.   Wash and trim the string beans, cut them in 1-inch pieces, and boil them in salted water until they are just tender— not a minute longer. Run cold water over them until they are

cool and put them in the refrigerator. Wash the watercress, trim off the heavy stems, and cut in half any very large pieces.

3.   Quarter and thinly slice the red onion. Peel and coarsely chop the hard-boiled eggs. Peel the cucumber, halve it lengthwise, and slice it.

4.   Clean the mushrooms, trim off the stems, and slice them thinly.

5.   Toss all the vegetable ingredients together in a bowl. Blend Sour Cream Dressing I with the mayonnaise; pour the dressing over the salad and toss again until everything is evenly coated.

Tomato Omelet
Servings: 6

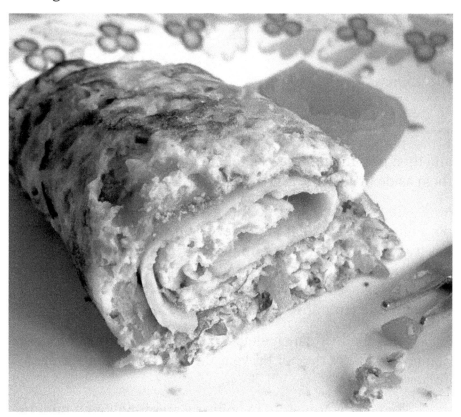

Ingredients:

8 medium sized tomatoes 2 cloves garlic

2 bay leaves

½ tsp. dried tarragon, crushed 1 tsp. salt, and more to taste 2 Tbs. chopped fresh parsley 1 medium-sized yellow onion 3 Tbs. olive oil

½ tsp. dried basil, crushed

5 cured black olives, pitted and sliced coarse ground black pepper to taste

8 to 10 eggs milk

Directions:

1.   Blanch the tomatoes in boiling water for about 2 minutes and then peel them. Chop the tomatoes very coarsely and put them aside in a bowl with the salt.

2.   Chop the onion, mince the garlic, and sauté them in the olive oil in a large skillet until they begin to show color. Add the bay leaves and sauté a few minutes more. Add the tomatoes, the basil, tarragon, parsley, and sliced olives, and cook over medium heat, stirring occasionally, until the sauce is thick. It should take about 40 to 45 minutes.

3.   Make individual omelets according to the directions. Spoon on some of the hot Provençale sauce just when the eggs are nearly set.

4.   Blanch the tomatoes in boiling water for about 2 minutes and then peel them. Chop the tomatoes very coarsely and put them aside in a bowl with the salt.

5.   Chop the onion, mince the garlic, and sauté them in the olive oil in a large skillet until they begin to show color. Add the bay leaves and sauté a few minutes more. Add the tomatoes, the basil, tarragon, parsley, and sliced olives, and cook over medium heat, stirring occasionally, until the sauce is thick. It should take about 40 to 45 minutes.

6.   Make individual omelets according to the directions. Spoon on some of the hot Provençale sauce just when the eggs are nearly set, and fold the omelets over the sauce. Serve.

Strawberry Marmalade

Servings: 3

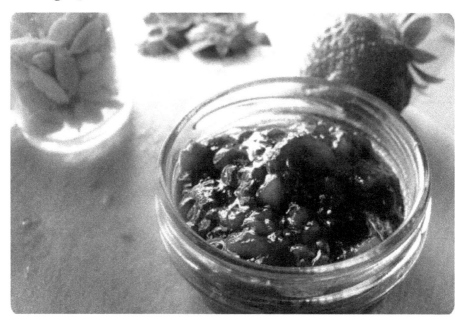

Ingredients:

600 grams of Sugar

1   kilogram of Strawberries.

Directions:

1.   Wash your strawberries. Cut into smaller sized pieces.

2.   Put your strawberries in a casserole dish and cover them in sugar.

3.   Let them sit overnight in order to get their juices extracted. This will turn your sugar into a red colored syrup.

4.   Put the casserole dish on a high heat and stir constantly until your sugar has dissolved and fruit has boiled.

5.   When it begins to foam, clean it using a spoon.

6.   Lower the heat and stir often for approximately 20 minutes. You

don't want marmalade sticking to the bottom.

7.   Take off heat when it is shiny and thick.

8.   Seal in jars in order to preserve. Good for up to a year.

9.   Serve and Enjoy!

Potato and Zucchini Omelet

Servings: 3

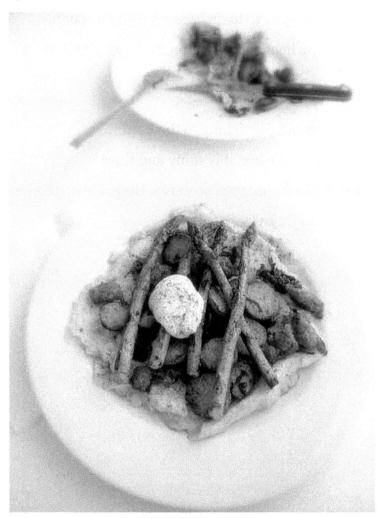

Ingredients:

½ lb. potato (about 1¼ cups diced)

½ lb. zucchini (about 1½ cups diced)

⅔ cup chopped onion (1 small) 1 Tbs. butter

2   Tbs. olive oil

¼ tsp. dried dill weed

¼ tsp. dried basil, crushed

½ tsp. crushed dried red pepper salt to taste

fresh-ground black pepper to taste 5 to 6 eggs

butter for frying garnish

sour cream

Directions:

1.   Peel or scrub the potato and cut it in ½-inch dice. Wash, trim, and finely dice the zucchini. Drop the diced potato into boiling salted water and cook for 5 minutes, then drain it and set it aside. Cook the diced zucchini in boiling water for 3 to 4 minutes, drain, and set aside.

2.   Heat the butter and the olive oil in a medium-sized skillet and sauté the onions in it until they start to color.

3.   Add the partially cooked potato and zucchini, the dill weed, basil, crushed red pepper, and salt. Cook this mixture over medium heat, stirring often, until the potatoes are just tender. Grind in some black pepper and add more salt if needed.

4.   Make either 2 medium-sized or 3 small omelets according to the directions. When the eggs are almost set, spoon some of the hot vegetables onto one side and fold the other side of the omelet over the filling. Slide the omelets out onto warm plates and serve immediately with sour cream.

Secret Breakfast Sundaes

Servings: 4

Ingredients:

6 slices of Bacon

1/2 cup of Heavy Whipping Cream

5 tablespoons of Pure Maple Syrup or Pancake Syrup

3 tablespoons of Light Brown Sugar

3/4 cup of Granola Cereal

2 cups of Coffee Ice Cream

2 cups of Butter Pecan Ice Cream

4 Fresh Strawberries

Directions:

1.   Preheat your oven to 400 degrees.

2.   Arrange your bacon on a non-stick baking sheet. Sprinkle 1/2 of your brown sugar over the bacon. Bake for approximately 6

minutes. Turn the bacon and sprinkle the remaining brown sugar over it. Bake for an additional 6 minutes until bacon is dark brown. Remove from your oven and allow to cool on a wire rack. Once your bacon has cooled, crumble it up and set it aside.

3.   Beat together a tablespoon of maple syrup with a 1/2 cup of cream in a 2-quart metal bowl using an electric mixer. Beat until stiff peaks form and then set aside.

4.   Spoon 2 tablespoons of granola into 4 parfait glasses. Evenly scoop the butter pecan ice cream into glasses and sprinkle them with your remaining granola. Add your coffee ice cream to each glass and evenly drizzle the remaining maple syrup on top. Sprinkle with your bacon, and top with strawberries.

5.   Serve and Enjoy!

Banana Nut Oatmeal

Servings: 1

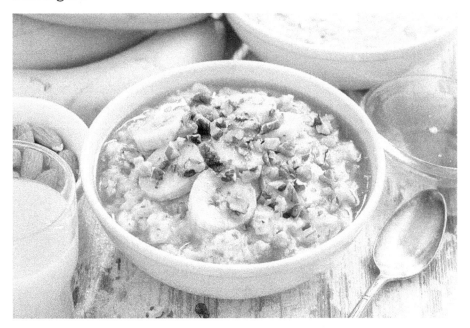

Ingredients:

1   Peeled Banana

1/2 cup of Skim Milk

1/4 cup of Quick Cooking Oats 3 tablespoons of Honey

2   tablespoons of Chopped Walnuts 1 teaspoon of Flax Seeds

Directions:

1.   Combine your milk, oats, honey, walnuts, banana, and
flax seeds in a microwave safe bowl. Cook in your microwave for
2 minutes on high. Mash your banana using a fork and stir it
into the mixture.

2.   Serve and Enjoy!

Greek Frittata w/ Zucchini, Tomatoes, Feta, and Herbs

Servings: 4

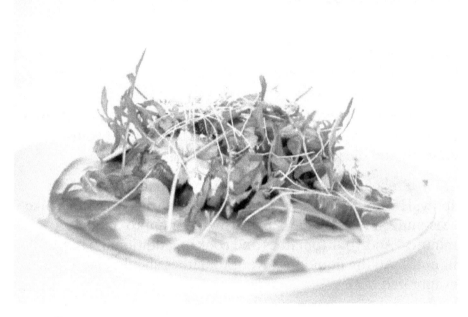

Ingredients:

6 Eggs

15 ounces of Diced Tomatoes

1 Diced Medium Zucchini

1 tablespoon of Olive Oil

2 cloves of Minced Garlic

1/2 cup of Mozzarella Cheese

1 tablespoon of Cream

1/4 cup of Crumbled Feta Cheese

1/4 teaspoon of Oregano

1/2 teaspoon of Dried Basil

1 teaspoon of Spike Seasoning

Cracked Black Pepper

Directions:

1.   Pour your tomatoes into your colander and allow them to drain out any liquid into your sink. Cut the ends off your zucchini and dice it into smaller pieces.

2.   Preheat your broiler. Spray a frying pan with cooking spray. Heat olive oil in your pan. Add the garlic, zucchini, spike seasoning, and dried herb. Saute them for approximately 3 minutes. Add your tomatoes and cook an additional 3 to 5 minutes. All the liquid from your tomatoes should be evaporated.

3.   While your vegetables are cooking, break your eggs in a bowl and beat them well. Pour your eggs into the pan with your vegetable mix and cook an additional 2 to 3 minutes. Eggs should just be beginning to set.

4.   Add half of your feta and mozzarella cheese. Stir them in gently. Cook approximately 3 minutes. Sprinkle the rest of your feta and mozzarella cheese over top and allow to cook for 3 more minutes with a lid covering your pan. Cheese should be mostly melted and the eggs should be nearly set.

5.   Place under your broiler until the top becomes browned slightly. Should only take a few minutes. Keep a close eye on it. Rotate the pan if necessary to get an even browning.

6.   Sprinkle any additional fresh herbs if you so desire. Cut into pie shaped wedges.

7.   Serve and Enjoy!

Greek Yogurt Pancakes

Servings: 4

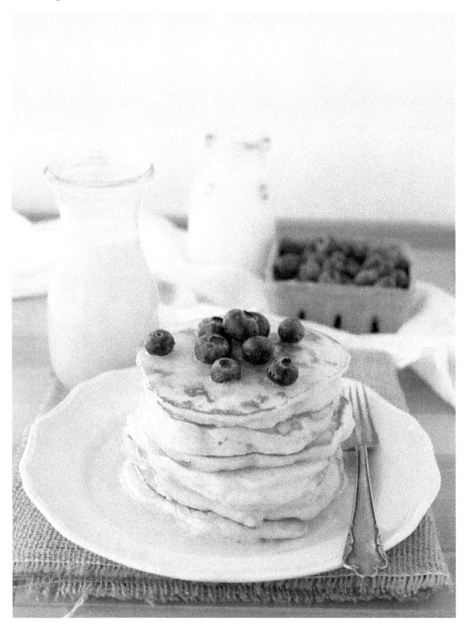

Ingredients:

One cup of Old-Fashioned Oats

2 tablespoons of Flax Seeds 1 teaspoon of Baking Soda

1/2 cup of All Purpose Flour

1/4 teaspoon of Salt

2   cups of Vanilla Greek Yogurt

2 tablespoons of Honey or Agave

2 Large Eggs

2 tablespoons of Canola Oil Syrup

Fresh Fruit

Directions:

1.   Combine oats, seeds, flour, baking soda, and salt in your blender and pulse for approximately 30 seconds.

2.   Add in your eggs, yogurt, agave, and oil. Blend until it is smooth. Let your batter stand approximately 20 minutes in order to thicken.

3.   Heat your skillet over a medium heat. Brush your skillet with oil. Ladle your batter 1/4 of a cup at a time into your skillet. Cook your pancakes until the bottoms turn golden brown and bubbles begin forming on top. Should take about 2 minutes. Turn over your pancakes and cook until the bottoms are golden brown. Should take another 2 minutes.

4.   Transfer pancakes to your baking sheet. Keep warm in your oven. Repeat process until all your batter is cooked.

5.   Add on desired syrup and fruit toppings.

6.   Serve and Enjoy!

Mediterranean Tofu Scramble

Servings: 4

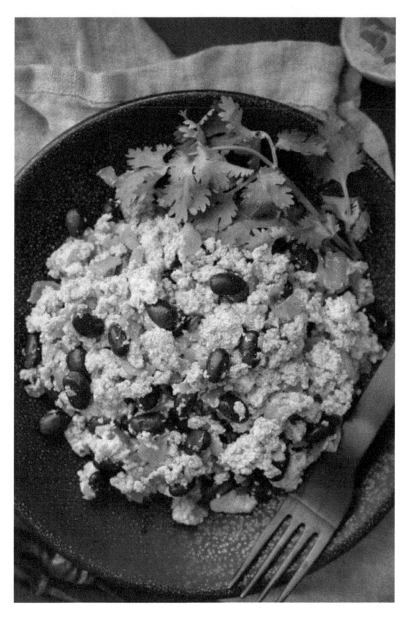

Ingredients:

2 tablespoons of Olive Oil

1 Diced Purple Onion

2 cloves of Minced Garlic

1 pound of Extra Firm Tofu

1 Diced Medium Red Bell Pepper

1 tablespoon of Lemon Juice

2 tablespoons of Soy Sauce

2 tablespoons of Seasoning

1 teaspoon of Ground Turmeric

1/4 cup of Finely Chopped Fresh Parsley

Directions:

3   Chopped Scallions

1/2 teaspoon of Red Pepper Flakes Toast

Hot Sauce Pita Bread Hummus

1.   Coat bottom of your large skillet with olive oil and put it over a medium heat. Once the oil is hot, add your onion and saute until it has softened. Should take about 5 minutes. Add your garlic and cook an additional minute.

2.   Crumble your tofu into your skillet and add your soy sauce, bell pepper, seasoning, lemon juice, and red pepper flakes. Keep cooking, flipping with your spatula, until your bell pepper pieces are crisp and tender. Should take about 5 minutes. Remove from the heat and fold in your scallions and parsley.

3.   Serve with pita, toast, hot sauce, and hummus. Enjoy!

CPSIA information can be obtained
at www.ICGtesting.com
Printed in the USA
BVHW091523180321
602886BV00003B/672